Po1

Fast Focus Study Guide

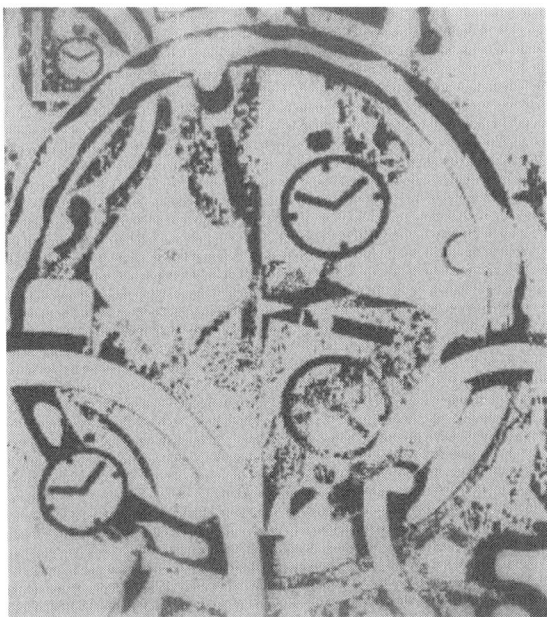

Acknowledgements

I dedicate this book to my beautiful wife and children, who I love more than all the water in all the oceans and all the seas.

CONTENTS

- This book is written for medical students, residents, and physicians who want to learn more about porphyria.

- Put this book in your bathroom or on your coffee table.

- This is a great resource for any medical professional.

- This Fast Focus Study Guide will provide you with a practical review of the key information you need to know.

- Buy this book now if you want this quick and concise information

Porphyria is a group of diseases related to a deficiency of one of the enzymes needed for heme synthesis.

There are of 8 different types of porphyria

We can separate types of porphyria into those that effect the skin, those that effect the nervous system and those that effect both the skin and the nervous system.

The types of porphyria that effect the skin include:

-Congenital erythropoietic porphyria

-Erythropoietic protoporphyria

-Hepatoerythropoietic porphyria

-Porphyria cutanea tarda

The types of porphyria that effect the nervous

system include:

-Acute intermittent porphyria

-ALAD deficiency porphyria

The types of porphyria that effects the skin

and nervous system include:

-Hereditary coproporphyria

-Variegate porphyria

We know that some types of porphyria are

more common than others.

Most Common	Porphyria cutanea tarda	→ 1 in 10,000
	Acute intermittent porphyria	→ 1 in 20,000
	Erythropoietic protoporphyria	→ 1 in 50,000 to 75,000
	Variegate porphyria	→ 1 in 100,000
	Hereditary Coproporphyria (HCP)	→ 2 in 1,000,000
	Congenital erythropoietic porphyria (CEP)	→ <1 in 1,000,000
	Hepatoerythropoietic porphyria	→ 100 cases reported
Least Common	ALAD-deficiency porphyria	→ 6 cases in literature

The 8 types of porphyria can be separated by frequency, separating the types of porphyria into those you are likely to see, those you are unlikely to see and those you will never likely to see.

The types of porphyria that are likely to be seen in a hematology practice (more common):

-Porphyria cutanea tarda (1 in 10,000)

-Acute intermittent porphyria (1 in 20,000)

-Erythropoietic protoporphyria (1 in 50,000-75,000)

The types of porphyria that are unlikely to be
diagnosed in clinical practice (less common):

-Variegate porphyria (1 in 100,000)

-Hereditary coproporphyria (HCP) (1 in
500,000)

-Congenital erythropoietic porphyria (CEP) (< 1
in 1,000,000)

The types of porphyria that a hematologist will probably never see in a lifetime (extremely rare):

-Hepatoerythropoietic porphyria (100 cases reported in literature)

-ALAD deficiency porphyria (6 cases in literature)

You Need To Know These Types of Porphyria Because They Are the Most Common:

-Porphyria Cutanea Tarda (Skin Blistering)

-Acute Intermittent Porphyria (Neuro-Visceral Symptoms)

-Erythropoietic Protoporphyria (Skin Blistering)

The Most Common Porphyria

Let us start with porphyria cutanea tarda (PCT) because it is the most common form of porphyria.

Which enzyme deficiency is responsible for porphyria cutanea tarda?

Uroporphyrinogen decarboxylase (UROD)

Is porphyria cutanea tarda inherited or acquired?

Most people with porphyria cutanea tarda have acquired the disease. In about 20% or less, it is inherited as an autosomal dominant trait.

How is porphyria cutanea tarda acquired?

Porphyria cutanea tarda is a hepatic porphyria. Therefore, many diseases that affect the liver can also lead to porphyria cutanea tarda. Some diseases associated with porphyria cutanea tarda include hepatitis, HIV, cirrhosis, hemochromatosis, and exogenous estrogen exposure.

What are the symptoms of porphyria cutanea tarda?

Porphyria cutanea tarda is typically characterized by blistering of sun exposed skin.

How do you diagnose porphyria cutanea
tarda?

First you have to suspect porphyria cutanea
tarda. Remember porphyria cutanea tarda
typically effects the skin. Remember
porphyria cutanea tarda can be acquired in
people with liver disease.

How do you diagnose porphyria cutanea tarda?

Next you will check a 24 hour urine. The urine Aminolevulinic acid level will be normal. The urine Porphobilinogen will be normal. The urine Uroporphyrin will be elevated

Next let us discuss Acute Intermittent Porphyria because it is the second most common form of porphyria.

Acute Intermittent Porphyria

- Affects women more than men, with a ratio of 2:1.

- Symptoms generally begin in adulthood at age 18-40 years.

- Most patients are completely free of symptoms between attacks.

Acute Intermittent Porphyria

-Course of the neurological manifestations is highly variable.

-Acute attacks of porphyria may resolve quite rapidly.

-Sudden death can occur.

Which enzyme deficiency is responsible for
acute intermittent porphyria?

A deficiency of porphobilinogen deaminase is
responsible for acute intermittent porphyria.

More information about acute intermittent porphyria!

- The enzyme deficiency alone is not enough to produce the symptoms of acute intermittent porphyria.

- Other activating factors such as drugs, hormones, and dietary changes are often present. Sometimes activating factors cannot be identified.

- Most people who have a mutation in the gene for AIP never develop symptoms; this is referred to as "latent" AIP

Which enzyme deficiency is responsible for
acute intermittent porphyria?

A deficiency of porphobilinogen deaminase is
responsible for acute intermittent porphyria.

Is acute intermittent porphyria inherited or acquired?

Acute intermittent porphyria is inherited in an autosomal dominant fashion.

What are the symptoms of acute intermittent porphyria?

When people have attacks, the symptoms are neuro-visceral without skin manifestations.

Other symptoms of acute intermittent porphyria?

-Vomiting and diarrhea

-Seizures, mental status changes, cortical blindness, and coma.

-Other symptoms include fever, hypertension and tachycardia.

What are the other symptoms of acute intermittent porphyria?

-Abdominal pain

-Psychiatric symptoms such as hysteria

-Peripheral neuropathy, mainly motor neuropathy.

-Constipation

-Colicky abdominal pain

How do you diagnose acute intermittent porphyria?

First you have to suspect acute intermit porphyria. Remember acute intermittent porphyria typically presents with neurovisceral symptoms. The symptoms are often characterized by abdominal pain which can sometimes be associated with nausea, vomiting, diarrhea, muscle weakness, confusion, and seizures.

How do you diagnose acute intermittent porphyria?

Check a spot urine for porphobilinogen (PBG). If the spot urine or 24 hour urine does not have elevated Porphobilinogen (PBG) then the patient does not have acute intermittent porphyria.

How do you diagnose acute intermittent porphyria?

If the testing is positive for spot urine for porphobilinogen (PBG). Then test for 5-aminolevulinic acid (urine), porphobilinogen deaminase (erythrocytes) and the 5-aminolevulinic acid (urine).

How do you diagnose acute intermittent porphyria?

In acute intermittent porphyria the 5-aminolevulinic acid (urine) will be elevated and the porphobilinogen deaminase (erythrocytes) will be normal.

Next we will discuss erythropoietic protoporphyria.

Erythropoietic protoporphia and X-linked protoporphia (XLP) are categorized together as the third most common types of porphyria. Symptoms usually first occur in early childhood.

Symptoms of erythropoietic porphyria include sun sensitivity characterized by severe pain and swelling of sun-exposed areas usually without blistering or scarring. This disease is characterized by elevations of protoporphyrin in the liver

Erythropoietic protoporphyria is caused by a deficiency of the enzyme, ferrochelatase (FECH).

Are erythropoietic protoporphia and X-linked protoporphia inherited or acquired?

These disorders are inherited. Erythropoietic protoporphia is an autosomal recessive disorder. X-linked protoporphia is inherited in an x-linked fashion.

What are the symptoms of erythropoietic protoporphia?

Painful photosensitivity sometimes even with indoor light exposure most often involving the face and the upper surfaces of the arms, hands, and feet and the exposed surfaces of the legs. Burning and itching sensation on the surface of the skin.

How do you diagnose erythropoietic protoporphia?

First you have to suspect erythropoietic protoporphia. Remember erythropoietic protoporphia often presents with skin sensitivity characterized by severe burning symptoms. These skin symptoms often are associated with erythema and swelling of the skin, but often without blisters.

How do you diagnose erythropoietic protoporphia?

Next you will check the total plasma porphyrins. If the patient has normal testing for total plasma porphyrins, they likely don't have porphyria that effects the skin.

How do you diagnose erythropoietic protoporphia?

The testing for total plasma porphyrins will be positive. To confirm this diagnosis, the serum protoporphyrin and the red blood cells erythrocyte free protoporphyrin will be elevated.

What will be the quickest porphyria screening test for a patient with acute neuro-visceral symptoms without skin symptoms?

Send a 24 hour urine for total porphyrins, urinary delta-aminolevulinic acid and porphobilinogen. If these are normal, the patient does not have a neuro-visceral porphyria.

Acute intermittent porphyria (the most common porphyria that causes neuro-visceral symptoms) and ALAD deficiency porphyria (6 cases in the literature) are among the different types of porphyria that present with neuro-visceral symptoms.

There are two additional types of porphyria that cause neuro-visceral symptoms, but these types of porphyria cause both skin and neuro-visceral symptoms. These types of porphyria are hereditary coproporphyria (1 in 100,000) and variegate porphyria (1 in 1,000,000 people).

The 4 types of porphyria cause neuro-visceral attacks include:

- Acute intermittent porphyria (most common)

- Hereditary coproporphyria

- Variegate porphyria

- Aminolevulinate dehydratase deficiency porphyria (extremely rare)

What will be the quickest porphyria screening test for a patient with skin symptoms without neuro-visceral symptoms?

You will check the total plasma porphyrins. If the patient has normal testing for total plasma porphyrins, they likely don't have porphyria that effects the skin.

Remember the types of porphyria that effect the skin:

- Porphyria cutanea tarda

- Congenital erythropoietic porphyria

- Hepatoerythropoietic porphyria

- Erythropoietic protoporphyria

Porphyria with skin symptoms

Porphyria cutanea tarda (most common) and erythropoietic protoporphyria (1 in 50,000 to 75,000) are the most common types of porphyria that present with skin symptoms. Congenital erythropoietic porphyria (<1 in 1,000,000) and Hepatoerythropoietic porphyria (100 cases reported) are uncommon.

Genetic testing can be done to confirm the diagnosis of porphyria with the exception of porphyria cutanea tarda (only 20% of porphyria cutanea tarda is genetic).

What is the genetic mutation associated with hereditary coproporphyria?

CPOX gene mutation

What is the genetic mutation associated with variegate porphyria?

PPOX gene mutation

What is the genetic mutation associated with congenital erythropoietic porphyria?

UROS gene mutation

What is the genetic mutation associated with

hepatoerythropoietic porphyria?

UROD gene mutation

Treating Porphyria Cutanea Tarda:

- Avoid alcohol

- Avoid sunlight

- Phlebotomy

Treating Acute Intermittent Porphyria:

- Pain control

- Rehydration

- Antiemetics

- IV/oral carbohydrates

- IV heme

- Supportive care

Treatment for Erythropoietic protoporphyria:

- Sunlight protection

- Beta-Carotene

- Vitamin D replacement

Treatment for Variegate Porphyria:

- Remove exacerbating factors

- Pain control

- Rehydration

- Antiemetics

- IV/oral carbohydrates

- IV heme

- Supportive care

Treatment for Hereditary Coproporphyria:

- Remove exacerbating factors

- Pain control

- Rehydration

- Antiemetics

- IV/oral carbohydrates

- IV heme

- Supportive care

Treatment for Congenital Erythropoietic:

Porphyria

- Blood transfusion

- Splenectomy

- Stem cell transplant

- Supportive care

Treatment for Hepatoerythropoietic porphyria:

- Avoid alcohol

- Avoid sunlight

- Phlebotomy

Treatment for ALAD-deficiency porphyria:

- Remove exacerbating factors

- Pain control

- Rehydration

- Antiemetics

- IV/oral carbohydrates

- IV heme

- Supportive care

Summary and Important Points

Remember there are 8 different types of porphyria. These can be divided into those we might see, those we are unlikely to see and those we will probably never seen.

The types of porphyria we are most likely to see:

1. Remember porphyria cutanea tarda

2. Remember acute intermittent porphyria

3. Remember erythropoietic protoporphia

Diagnose porphyria cutanea tarda:

-Check a 24 hour urine

-The urine Aminolevulinic acid level will be normal

-The urine Porphobilinogen will be normal

-The urine Uroporphyrin will be elevated

Diagnose erythropoietic protoporphia:

Testing for total plasma porphyrins will be positive. To confirm this diagnosis, the serum protoporphyrin and the red blood cells erythrocyte free protoporphyrin will be elevated.

Summary and Important Points

1. Remember what to think when a patient presents with neuro-visceral symptoms

2. Remember what to think when a patient presents with skin symptoms

What will be the quickest porphyria screening test for a patient with acute neuro-visceral symptoms without skin symptoms?

1. Send a 24 hour urine for total porphyrins, Urinary delta-aminolevulinic acid and porphobilinogen.

2. If these are normal, the patient does not have a neuro-visceral porphyria

What will be the quickest porphyria screening test for a patient with skin symptoms without neuro-visceral symptoms?

1. You will check the total plasma porphyrins.

2. If the patient has normal testing for total plasma porphyrins, they likely don't have porphyria that effects the skin.

This concludes Porphyria: Fast Focus Study
Guide

Search Amazon Kindle books to find other study
guides written by

JT Thomas, MD

Internal Medicine Study Guide

Hematology Study Guide

Medical Oncology Study Guide

Rheumatology Study Guide

21970423R00043

Printed in Great Britain
by Amazon